Migraine Tracker Journal

A 3-Month Migraine Logbook for Tracking Symptoms, Food, Mood, and Medication to Discover Triggers and Patterns

Book & Bat Publishing

Copyright

ISBN 978-1-923500-14-3

First edition, 2025

Book and Bat Publishing

PO Box 820, Indooroopilly, QLD 4068, Australia

info@bookandbat.com

Disclaimer

This tracker is not a medical tool and does not provide medical advice. It is intended for personal use, education, and reflection only. The information included is general in nature and may not apply to your individual situation.

Always consult a qualified healthcare professional before making decisions about your health, diagnosis, or treatment. Do not delay, disregard, or change medical advice because of anything you read in this book.

The author and publisher have made every effort to ensure accuracy but make no guarantees and accept no responsibility for errors or omissions. By using this tracker, you agree that the author and publisher are not liable for any loss, harm, or damages of any kind arising from its use.

Contents

Welcome to Your 3-Month Migraine Tracker

Migraines are hard to live with. Tracking what affects how often they occur, and how intense they are, can make a real difference to your quality of life. Whether you've had migraines for years or are just beginning to explore the causes of your symptoms, this tracker can help you gather clear, useful information.

It can help you notice patterns, understand your symptoms, and see what brings relief. It can also give your doctor useful information to guide treatment.

The international Classification of Headache Disorders (ICHD-3) and most clincians recommend tracking for three months to establish whether a pattern or change is consistent. This tracker can help you spot trends, like food triggers, hormone shifts, or weather changes, without feeling too overwhelming. It balances detail with manageability.

Migraine Can Look Different for Everyone

Some people experience visual changes (aura), dizziness, or even speech problems. Others may have chronic migraine, with symptoms on more days than not. This tracker can help you notice your own patterns, no matter the type.

A blank tracker and key are included so you can track anything else that's important to you, such as symptoms, triggers, or new treatments.

What Is a Migraine?

A migraine is much more than "just a headache." It's a neurological condition that affects nearly 40 million Americans and one billion people worldwide (American Migraine Foundation, 2023).

While a regular headache can cause discomfort, migraines often involve:

- Moderate to severe pain, usually on one side of the head
- Throbbing or pulsing pain
- Blurred vision or visual disturbances (aura)
- Dizziness or feeling faint
- Nausea or vomiting
- Sensitivity to light, sound, or smells
- Symptoms that interfere with daily activities
- Episodes lasting from several hours to several days

Migraines are believed to involve changes in brain chemicals and blood vessels, with genetics playing a significant role. If you have a family member with migraines, you're more likely to experience them too.

The Four Stages of a Migraine

Not everyone experiences each stage, and your own symptoms may look different from the examples here. These stages are a guide to help you notice which parts of the migraine cycle apply to you.

1. Prodrome (Before the Pain)

This early warning phase can begin hours or even days before the headache starts. Common prodrome signs:

- Mood changes (irritability, depression, or unusual excitement)
- Food cravings
- Yawning excessively
- Neck stiffness
- Increased thirst or urination
- Difficulty concentrating

Recognizing your prodrome symptoms can give you time to take medication or avoid triggers before the pain begins.

2. Aura (Warning Phase)

About 25-30% of people with migraines experience aura symptoms. This phase usually lasts 20-60 minutes before the headache starts. Aura may include:

- Visual disturbances (flashing lights, zigzag lines, blind spots)
- Numbness or tingling, usually in the face or hands
- Difficulty speaking
- Weakness on one side of the body
- Hearing noises or music

If you experience severe weakness, confusion, or trouble speaking that doesn't resolve quickly, seek medical attention immediately. These can be signs of a stroke.

3. Headache Phase

This is when the typical migraine pain occurs. This phase can last from 4 hours to 3 days without treatment. Characteristics include:

- Throbbing or pulsing pain, often on one side of the head (it can affect both sides)
- Pain that worsens with movement, light, or sound
- Nausea and vomiting
- Dizziness or lightheadedness
- Extreme sensitivity to stimuli (lights, sounds, smells).

4. Postdrome (Recovery Phase)

After the headache passes, you may experience the "migraine hangover." This phase can last 24-48 hours.

Postdrome symptoms include:

- Feeling drained or washed out or mood changes
- Mild confusion or difficulty concentrating
- Head pain when suddenly moving
- Continued sensitivity to light and sound.

Common Migraine Triggers

Triggers vary widely among individuals. Not every trigger can be avoided, but recognizing yours can make day-to-day life easier. Sometimes patterns only appear when triggers combine, like lack of sleep plus certain foods.

Awareness helps reduce your overall migraine load and gives you a clearer sense of what to plan for.

Not all of these will apply to you, and you don't need to track every single one. The trackers in this book focus on the factors most commonly linked to migraine, so you can start with those and add others if you notice a personal pattern.

Your personal triggers might include:

Environmental Factors

- Weather changes or barometric pressure shifts
- Bright or flickering lights
- Strong smells (perfumes, cleaning products)
- Loud noises
- Smoke

Lifestyle Factors

- Irregular sleep patterns (too much or too little sleep)
- Skipped meals or fasting
- Dehydration
- Stress or stress letdown after a stressful period
- Intense physical activity

Dietary Factors

- Alcohol (especially red wine)
- Caffeine (too much or withdrawal)
- Aged cheeses
- Processed foods with nitrates
- Artificial sweeteners
- Chocolate (for some people)

Hormonal Factors

- Menstrual cycle fluctuations
- Hormonal birth control
- Pregnancy or menopause

- Hormone replacement therapy
- Changes in testosterone levels

Other Common Triggers

- Certain medications
- Neck tension or poor posture
- Eye strain
- Travel, jet lag, changes in altitude or routine

Rebound Headaches

Rebound (also called medication-overuse headache) can happen when pain relief medications are taken too often. Tracking your medication use alongside migraine days can help you and your doctor see whether this might be part of your pattern.

How to Use This Tracker

This 3-month tracker will help you identify patterns in your migraines by tracking:

- Your daily habits and potential triggers
- Detailed information about each migraine episode
- Treatments you've tried and their effectiveness

For best results:

- Fill out the tracker consistently, even on good days
- Complete a migraine episode page as soon as possible after an attack
- Bring this tracker to doctor appointments
- Review the monthly summary pages to look for patterns

There are also trackers to help you identify triggers you may not be aware of yet. You don't need to use all the trackers, only the one/s that are relevant.

Remember that managing migraines is often about finding small improvements that add up over time. By tracking your experiences, you're taking an active role in your health management.

You may not see clear patterns right away. That's normal. Even small notes, like a tick here or there, build up over time to give you useful insights. Don't worry if you miss a day, just keep going. The value comes from the bigger picture, not from perfection.

A Note About Medical Care

This tracker is not a medical tool and does not provide medical advice. It is designed to help you notice patterns and prepare for conversations with your healthcare provider.

Always consult a qualified medical professional about your symptoms, diagnosis, and treatment. Do not ignore or delay seeking professional advice because of anything you record or read in this book. Please contact your healthcare provider if:

- your migraine pattern changes,
- you experience new or severe symptoms, or
- treatments stop working.

If you ever experience sudden, severe, or unusual symptoms (such as weakness, confusion, or vision changes that do not resolve quickly), seek medical attention immediately.

It's time to start tracking and taking control of your migraine journey!

If you find this tracker helpful, please consider leaving a short review. Reviews make it easier for others with migraines to discover tools that might support them too.

My Migraine Profile

Baseline & Quick Reference

Start here to set your direction and record what you already know. This page creates your baseline and serves as a quick reference for appointments. Complete your profile first to give yourself a clear starting point, then update it as patterns shift or you try new treatments. Your profile helps you compare what you knew at the start with what you learn along the way.

TIMING

Tracker Start Date: / / 20 Expected End Date: / / 20

GOALS FOR THIS TRACKER PERIOD

Start by defining your aims. This helps you use the tracker with purpose and gives you something clear to measure.

- ☐ Reduce frequency
- ☐ Reduce severity
- ☐ Identify new triggers
- ☐ Try new treatments
- ☐ Improve recovery time
- ☐ Better sleep patterns
- ☐ Other:

MY TYPICAL MIGRAINE PATTERN

Start by defining your aims. This helps you use the tracker with purpose and gives you something clear to measure.

Warning signs I usually notice

Typical duration

Most effective relief strategies

When I usually take medication

CURRENT MEDICATIONS

Preventive treatments (daily/regular medications)

Acute/rescue treatments (taken during migraine)

Most effective relief strategies

When I usually take medication

MY EMERGENCY PLAN

When to contact my doctor

When to seek emergency care

Who to contact for help

OTHER HEALTH CONDITIONS

List any other health conditions, medications, or factors that might relate to your migraines.

Tip: You can update this profile at any time as you learn more about your migraine patterns. Bring this page to doctor appointments as a quick reference.

Health Care Visits

Healthcare visits can blur together, especially when you are managing frequent migraines or seeing more than one provider. These pages give you a structured place to record the essentials to help you create a reliable record over time.

Date	Provider Name & Role

Location & Contact Details ______________________________

____

Reason for Visit ______________________________

____

Questions to Ask

____

____

____

____

____

____

____

Outcomes / Next Steps

Treatments recommended ______________________________

____

____

____

____

____

Tests / referrals ______________________________

____

____

____

____

____

____

Follow-up date ______________________________

Health Care Visits

Healthcare visits can blur together, especially when you are managing frequent migraines or seeing more than one provider. These pages give you a structured place to record the essentials to help you create a reliable record over time.

Date	Provider Name & Role

Location & Contact Details ______________________________

____

Reason for Visit ______________________________

____

Questions to Ask

____

____

____

____

____

____

____

Outcomes / Next Steps

Treatments recommended ______________________________

____

____

____

____

____

Tests / referrals ______________________________

____

____

____

____

____

____

Follow-up date ______________________________

Health Care Visits

Healthcare visits can blur together, especially when you are managing frequent migraines or seeing more than one provider. These pages give you a structured place to record the essentials to help you create a reliable record over time.

Date	Provider Name & Role

Location & Contact Details ______________________________

____

Reason for Visit ______________________________

____

Questions to Ask

____

____

____

____

____

____

____

Outcomes / Next Steps

Treatments recommended ______________________________

____

____

____

____

____

Tests / referrals ______________________________

____

____

____

____

____

____

Follow-up date ______________________________

Health Care Visits

Healthcare visits can blur together, especially when you are managing frequent migraines or seeing more than one provider. These pages give you a structured place to record the essentials to help you create a reliable record over time.

Date	Provider Name & Role

Location & Contact Details ______________________________

____

Reason for Visit ______________________________

____

Questions to Ask

____

____

____

____

____

____

____

Outcomes / Next Steps

Treatments recommended ______________________________

____

____

____

____

____

Tests / referrals ______________________________

____

____

____

____

____

____

Follow-up date ______________________________

Health Care Visits

Healthcare visits can blur together, especially when you are managing frequent migraines or seeing more than one provider. These pages give you a structured place to record the essentials to help you create a reliable record over time.

Date	Provider Name & Role

Location & Contact Details ____________________

____

Reason for Visit ____________________

____

Questions to Ask

____

____

____

____

____

____

____

Outcomes / Next Steps

Treatments recommended ____________________

____

____

____

____

____

Tests / referrals ____________________

____

____

____

____

____

____

Follow-up date ____________________

Health Care Visits

Healthcare visits can blur together, especially when you are managing frequent migraines or seeing more than one provider. These pages give you a structured place to record the essentials to help you create a reliable record over time.

Date	Provider Name & Role

Location & Contact Details ____________________

____

Reason for Visit ____________________

____

Questions to Ask

____

____

____

____

____

____

____

Outcomes / Next Steps

Treatments recommended ____________________

____

____

____

____

____

Tests / referrals ____________________

____

____

____

____

____

____

Follow-up date ____________________

Health Care Visits

Healthcare visits can blur together, especially when you are managing frequent migraines or seeing more than one provider. These pages give you a structured place to record the essentials to help you create a reliable record over time.

Date	Provider Name & Role

Location & Contact Details ______________________________

____

Reason for Visit ______________________________

____

Questions to Ask

____

____

____

____

____

____

____

Outcomes / Next Steps

Treatments recommended ______________________________

____

____

____

____

____

Tests / referrals ______________________________

____

____

____

____

____

____

Follow-up date ______________________________

Health Care Visits

Healthcare visits can blur together, especially when you are managing frequent migraines or seeing more than one provider. These pages give you a structured place to record the essentials to help you create a reliable record over time.

Date	Provider Name & Role

Location & Contact Details ____________________

____

Reason for Visit ____________________

____

Questions to Ask

____

____

____

____

____

____

____

Outcomes / Next Steps

Treatments recommended ____________________

____

____

____

____

____

Tests / referrals ____________________

____

____

____

____

____

____

Follow-up date ____________________

Health Care Visits

Healthcare visits can blur together, especially when you are managing frequent migraines or seeing more than one provider. These pages give you a structured place to record the essentials to help you create a reliable record over time.

Date	Provider Name & Role

Location & Contact Details ______________________________

____

Reason for Visit ______________________________

____

Questions to Ask

____

____

____

____

____

____

____

Outcomes / Next Steps

Treatments recommended ______________________________

____

____

____

____

____

Tests / referrals ______________________________

____

____

____

____

____

____

Follow-up date ______________________________

Health Care Visits

Healthcare visits can blur together, especially when you are managing frequent migraines or seeing more than one provider. These pages give you a structured place to record the essentials to help you create a reliable record over time.

Date	Provider Name & Role

Location & Contact Details ______________________

____

Reason for Visit ______________________

____

Questions to Ask

____

____

____

____

____

____

____

Outcomes / Next Steps

Treatments recommended ______________________

____

____

____

____

____

Tests / referrals ______________________

____

____

____

____

____

____

Follow-up date ______________________

Section 1. Core Tracking

According to the National Headache Foundation (2022), patients who keep headache diaries often have better outcomes when working with their healthcare providers to develop treatment plans. This section forms the foundation of your tracker. It brings together the monthly calendars for the "big picture" and the focused trackers that help you zoom in on specific areas linked with migraine.

How To Use These Pages

The **monthly calendars** give you a quick, at-a-glance view of migraine days, severity, and the everyday factors that may connect with them. Filling them in daily, even on good days, builds a reliable overview of your migraine activity. A simple 0 for severity, or leaving the box blank, still provides valuable information because it shows when migraines did not occur.

The **focused trackers** let you explore common migraine influences in more detail, including sleep, food and hydration, stress and emotions, hormones, and medication or supplement use. Two blank trackers are included for anything unique to you. These pages help you see how particular factors may connect with your migraine days.

Perfection Not Required

You do not need to be perfect. Partial notes are still valuable. The goal is to notice patterns over time, not to keep flawless records. Many people find that several small factors add up until they cross a personal threshold, like pressure building until it tips over. Tracking helps you see the bigger picture of how those factors combine.

Ratings Scales

Throughout this tracker, you'll see two similar scales:

- Migraine severity: 0–5, where 0 = no migraine and 5 = severe.
- All other ratings: 1–5, where 1 = minimal and 5 = very high.

Do Your Own Research

Migraine research is always developing, and new insights appear regularly.

If you want to explore more, try searching with terms such as *migraine food triggers*, *weather and migraine*, *migraine sleep patterns*, *new migraine research* or *new migraine treatments*.

Bringing your own questions and findings to your doctor can make these conversations more effective.

Monthly Migraine Trackers

Month 1: Example 20______

	Day 1	2	3	4	5	6	7	8	9	10	11	12	13	14	15	16	17	18	19	20	21	22	23	24	25	26	27	28	29	30	31
Severity	0	0	0	0	0	0	0	0	0	0	0	0	0	2	1	0	0	0	0	0	0	0	0	0	0	4	3	2	3	1	0
Treatment														R1	O1											R1	O	R1	O		
Effect														P	S											F	S	S*	S		
Sleep Issues															✓														✓		
Stress/Emotion														✓												✓	✓	✓			
Food/Diet														✓												✓	✓	✓			
Menstrual																										✓	✓	✓	✓	✓	
Weather													4P												5S			3H			
Exercise	2	2	2	2	4	1	0	2	2	2	2	4		1	2	2	2	2	4	1		2	2	2	5	2			1	2	2

Migraine Days 5 Medication Days 4 Avg Severity 2

Days with: Stress 6 Food/diet 5 Menstrual 5

MEDICATION CODES EXAMPLES

1. R1 – [Prescription medication name]
2. R2 - [Prescription medication name]
3. O1 – [OTC medication1 name]
4. O2 – [OTC medication2 name]
5. O3 - [OTC medication3 name]

KEY

- Severity Scale: 0 = no pain, 5 = severe
- Treatment Effect: 1 = no effect 5 = complete relief
- Sleep Issues: 1 = Slept well 5 = Broken sleep / poor quality
- Stress/Emotion: 1 = calm/stable 5 = very high/extreme
- Food/Diet: ate food commonly linked with migraine
- Weather: 1 = stable 5 = extreme. Optional: S storm, P pressure change, H heat/heatwave, C cold/sudden drop, W wind
- Exercise: 1 = no activity, 5 = very intense exercise

Month 1

Monthly Migraine Trackers

Month 1: ____________________ 20______

	Day 1	2	3	4	5	6	7	8	9	10	11	12	13	14	15	16	17	18	19	20	21	22	23	24	25	26	27	28	29	30	31
Severity																															
Treatment																															
Effect																															
Sleep Issues																															
Stress/Emotion																															
Food/Diet																															
Menstrual																															
Weather																															
Exercise																															

Migraine Days ______ Medication Days______ Avg Severity _____

Days with: Stress_____ Food/diet ______________ Menstrual _______

MEDICATION CODES

1. ______________________________
2. ______________________________
3. ______________________________
4. ______________________________
5. ______________________________

KEY

- Severity Scale: 0 = no pain, 5 = severe
- Treatment Effect: 1 = no effect 5 = complete relief
- Sleep Issues: 1 = Slept well 5 = Broken sleep / poor quality
- Stress/Emotion: 1 = calm/stable 5 = very high/extreme
- Food/Diet: ate food commonly linked with migraine
- Weather: 1 = stable 5 = extreme. Optional: S storm, P pressure change, H heat/heatwave, C cold/sudden drop, W wind
- Exercise: 1 = no activity, 5 = very intense exercise

Monthly Food & Hydration Tracker

Month 1: ________________ **20**______

Check if you consumed common trigger foods. Track water intake and note any suspected reactions. If you do not know if you have any food triggers, track your daily food consumption using the pages at the end of this set. Track the 8oz water cups per day on the last row.

Day	1	2	3	4	5	6	7	8	9	10	11	12	13	14	15	16	17	18	19	20	21	22	23	24	25	26	27	28	29	30	31
Caffeine																															
Alcohol																															
Processed Food																															
Fermented Food																															
Dairy																															
Chocolate																															
Citrus																															
Water Cups																															

Suspected Reactions____

____

____

____

____

Monthly Sleep Tracker

Month 1: ____________________ **20**______

Use the sleep quality scale to record your sleep hours and quality. Note any disruptions.

Day	1	2	3	4	5	6	7	8	9	10	11	12	13	14	15	16	17	18	19	20	21	22	23	24	25	26	27	28	29	30	31
Sleep Quality																															
Bedtime																															
Wake Time																															
Trouble falling asleep Y/N																															
# times awake																															
Meds/Supps																															
Naps																															

Sleep Quality Scale

1. Poor: Restless, multiple awakenings
2. Fair: Some tossing/turning, a few awakenings
3. Average: Generally restful with minor disruptions
4. Good: Solid sleep, woke feeling somewhat refreshed
5. Excellent: Deep sleep, woke feeling completely refreshed

Medications/Supplements Key

Example - Melatonin: M

Monthly Stress & Emotional Tracker

Month 1: ____________________ **20**______

Each day, mark your stress level (1–5, with 5 being most intense), tick any emotions you felt, add an asterisk (*) if you had a migraine, and record stress relief using the codes below

Day	1	2	3	4	5	6	7	8	9	10	11	12	13	14	15	16	17	18	19	20	21	22	23	24	25	26	27	28	29	30	31
Stress level																															
Anxious																															
Sad																															
Angry																															
Worried																															
Calm																															
Happy																															
Tired																															
Overwhelmed																															
Stress Relief																															

Key For Stress Relief Activities

Deep breathing (D)
Walking (W)
Reading (R)
Bath/shower (B)
Meditation (M)
Exercise (E)
Socializing (S)
Music (C)
Other (O): ____________

Biggest stressors this month were: ____________________

____

Stress relief that worked best and when was: ____________________

I noticed migraines most often when I felt: ____________________

Menstrual Cycle Tracker

Month 1: ______________ 20_____

Many people with migraine notice changes around their menstrual cycle. Attacks are most likely to occur in the days just before and just after a period begins, sometimes called the menstrual migraine window. For some, migraines also appear with ovulation, spotting, or during heavier flow.

Tracking your cycle alongside migraine activity can help show patterns that may otherwise be hard to spot.

If you are perimenopausal or postmenopausal, you may find the monthly or episodic trackers more useful for noticing patterns.

Day	1	2	3	4	5	6	7	8	9	10	11	12	13	14	15	16	17	18	19	20	21	22	23	24	25	26	27	28	29	30	31
Period Day																															
Flow																															
Ovulation																															
Symptoms																															
Other																															

Start at Cycle Day 1 on the first day of bleeding and number forward until your next period begins. Tick or shade boxes for Period Days, Spotting, and Other Symptoms as needed. Use the Flow codes below to record daily flow.

Key For Symptoms

Migraine (*)	Tender breasts (T)
Headache (H)	Nausea / GI changes (N)
Cramps (C)	Sleep changes (S)
Bloating (B)	Hot flush/night sweat (X)
Fatigue/Tiredness (F)	Other ( ):
Mood changes (M)	

Note any hormonal treatments, or natural hormonal changes affecting your migraines. Even small shifts can sometimes change migraine patterns:

____

____

____

Monthly Medication & Supplement Tracker

Month 1: ________________ 20_____

Write your medications and supplements in the key below (include dose). Each row is one medication/supplement. Tick on the days you take it. If you take more than once a day, add a tick for each dose. Use the notes section for side effects, missed doses, or anything unusual.

Meds/Supp	1	2	3	4	5	6	7	8	9	10	11	12	13	14	15	16	17	18	19	20	21	22	23	24	25	26	27	28	29	30	31

Key For Medications and Supplements

1. ____________
2. ____________
3. ____________
4. ____________
5. ____________
6. ____________
7. ____________
8. ____________
9. ____________
10. ____________

Notes

____

____

____

____

____

Monthly Tracker ____________________

Month: ____________ 20____

Track anything that is unique to you. Use the key and notes below to customize the tracker to suit.

	1	2	3	4	5	6	7	8	9	10	11	12	13	14	15	16	17	18	19	20	21	22	23	24	25	26	27	28	29	30	31

Key

Notes

Monthly Tracker ____________________

Month: ______________ 20____

Track anything that is unique to you. Use the key and notes below to customize the tracker to suit.

	1	2	3	4	5	6	7	8	9	10	11	12	13	14	15	16	17	18	19	20	21	22	23	24	25	26	27	28	29	30	31

Key

Notes

Monthly Tracker ____________________ Month: ______________ 20_____

Track anything that is unique to you. Use the key and notes below to customize the tracker to suit.

	1	2	3	4	5	6	7	8	9	10	11	12	13	14	15	16	17	18	19	20	21	22	23	24	25	26	27	28	29	30	31

Key

Notes

Food Tracking

About Food and Migraine

Food can be one of the factors that influence migraine. People react differently, and it is not always a single food that plays a role. For some, the issue is a combination of foods eaten together, for example cheese + red wine. For others it is the amount, the timing of meals, or specific additives.

Commonly reported triggers include caffeine, alcohol, chocolate, citrus, dairy, processed foods, and products with artificial sweeteners or preservatives. Brands can vary: one brand of cheddar might be fine, but another might be a trigger. Hidden ingredients such as creamers or flavorings may also matter.

Meal timing can be important. Skipping meals, eating later than usual, or having certain foods in the evening rather than earlier in the day *may* change how your body responds.

Crossing the Threshold

Migraines are often described as a *threshold condition*. Small factors build up until the level is high enough to bring on an attack.

Food can add to this load, sometimes in combination with stress, sleep changes, or hormones.

This Is an Experiment

This four-week journal is a good starting point. If you don't see patterns after the first month, consider continuing with a second set of trackers. This book includes two sets, so you can keep going if needed. Some foods are only eaten occasionally, or they act in combination with other triggers. Longer tracking gives you more chances to notice these links.

It is important to record every item you eat or drink as accurately as possible, including small snacks, drinks, and brand details. This is not about judging your diet. It is about being frank and honest so you can see the whole picture and understand where your threshold may be.

Use this tracker to record what you eat and drink, including brands, snacks, additives, and the time of day. If you get a migraine, add a star * on the day you get a migraine. This will help you compare with your migraine calendar to help you notice if patterns emerge.

EXAMPLE: Week 1 Food & Drink Journal

Date / /20________

Food	Sunday	Monday	Tuesday	Wednesday	Thursday	Friday	Saturday
Breakfast	Two eggs scrambled, wholegrain toast, black coffee (no sugar)	Oatmeal with milk [brand 1], sliced banana, green tea	Greek yogurt [brand 1], granola [brand 1], orange	Smoothie (spinach, banana, yogurt [brand 2]), water	Omelette (2 eggs, cheddar cheese [brand 1], tomato), black coffee	Wholegrain cereal [brand 1], milk [brand 1], black coffee	Pancakes (3 small, maple syrup), herbal tea
Morning Snack	Apple, plain water	Rice cakes [brand 1] with peanut butter, black coffee	Small chocolate bar [brand 1], water	Grapes, sparkling water	Pear, diet soda (with sweetener [brand 1])	Handful of almonds, black tea	Orange, plain water
Lunch	Turkey sandwich (deli meat [brand 1], cheddar [brand 2], lettuce, mayo [brand 1]), water	Salad (chicken breast, mixed greens, vinaigrette [brand 1]), wholegrain roll, water	Spaghetti with marinara sauce [brand 1], parmesan cheese [brand 1], water	Ham and cheese sandwich (ham [brand 2], cheddar [brand 1], mustard [brand 1]), water	Lentil soup [brand 1], bread roll, black coffee	Sushi roll (salmon, avocado), soy sauce [brand 1], green tea	Grilled chicken wrap (chicken breast, tortilla [brand 1], lettuce, mayo [brand 2]), water
Afternoon Snack	Yogurt [brand 2], plain water	Trail mix (nuts, raisins, chocolate pieces), ginger tea	Banana, sparkling water	Packet of chips [brand 1], plain water	Greek yogurt [brand 1], berries, plain water	Crackers [brand 1] with cheddar [brand 3], water	Handful of pretzels [brand 1], lemon tea

Food	Sunday	Monday	Tuesday	Wednesday	Thursday	Friday	Saturday
Dinner	Baked salmon, roasted vegetables, brown rice, chamomile tea	Chicken stir fry (chicken breast, vegetables, soy sauce [brand 2]), plain water	Beef stew (beef, carrots, potatoes, gravy [brand 1]), plain water	Spaghetti with meatballs (ground beef [brand 1], marinara [brand 2], parmesan [brand 2]), red wine (1 glass)	Grilled pork chop, mashed potato, broccoli, peppermint tea	Vegetarian pizza (cheese [brand 1], tomato sauce [brand 3], mixed vegetables), plain water	Roast chicken, roasted potatoes, green beans, black tea
Evening Snack	Small piece of dark chocolate [brand 2], plain water	Popcorn [brand 1], chamomile tea	Apple, chamomile tea	Cheese and crackers (cheddar [brand 4], crackers [brand 2]), plain water	Biscuit [brand 1], sleepy tea	Small slice of cheesecake [brand 1], plain water	Bowl of ice cream [brand 1], chamomile tea
Drinks	8 cups water, 1 black coffee, 1 ginger tea	7 cups water, 2 black coffees, 1 green tea	8 cups water, 1 black coffee, 1 sparkling water	7 cups water, 1 black coffee, 1 sparkling water, 1 glass red wine	8 cups water, 2 black coffees	7 cups water, 1 black coffee, 1 green tea, 1 herbal tea	8 cups water, 1 herbal tea

Suspected reactions or patterns noticed: ______________________________

Foods or drinks I noticed before migraine symptoms: ______________________________

Patterns or combinations that stood out: ______________________________

Notes for comparison with migraine calendar: ______________________________

How to Spot a Possible Food Trigger

- Look for timing. Migraine symptoms may appear within a few hours of eating, but sometimes the link shows up the next day. Compare what you ate in the 24–48 hours before an attack.
- Check for repetition. If the same food or drink shows up before more than one attack, note it. For example, if you notice migraines after both weekends where you had red wine, mark it as something to watch.
- Notice combinations. Some foods may only be a problem when eaten together, or when layered with other triggers like stress or lack of sleep. Cheese on its own may be fine, but cheese with wine may tip you over.
- Think about quantity. A small amount of a food may not cause issues, while larger portions might. One piece of chocolate may be fine, but several pieces could make a difference.
- Use your calendar. Compare your food journal with your migraine calendar to see which, if any, days line up.

Remember, a single episode is not enough to confirm a trigger. You are looking for patterns that repeat over time.

Important Note

This tracker is a tool for observation. If you notice possible food triggers, whether individual items or combinations, discuss them with a medical professional as part of your overall treatment plan.

Week 1 Food & Drink Journal

Date / /20______

Food	Sunday	Monday	Tuesday	Wednesday	Thursday	Friday	Saturday
Breakfast							
Morning Snack							
Lunch							
Afternoon Snack							

Food	Sunday	Monday	Tuesday	Wednesday	Thursday	Friday	Saturday
Dinner							
Evening Snack							
Drinks							

Suspected reactions or patterns: ______________________________

Food/drink before migraine symptoms: ______________________________

Patterns or combinations that stood out: ______________________________

Comparison with migraine calendar: ______________________________

Week 2 Food & Drink Journal

Date / /20______

Food	Sunday	Monday	Tuesday	Wednesday	Thursday	Friday	Saturday
Breakfast							
Morning Snack							
Lunch							
Afternoon Snack							

Food	Sunday	Monday	Tuesday	Wednesday	Thursday	Friday	Saturday
Dinner							
Evening Snack							
Drinks							

Suspected reactions or patterns: ____________________

Food/drink before migraine symptoms: ____________________

Patterns or combinations that stood out: ____________________

Comparison with migraine calendar: ____________________

Week 3 Food & Drink Journal

Date / /20______

Food	Sunday	Monday	Tuesday	Wednesday	Thursday	Friday	Saturday
Breakfast							
Morning Snack							
Lunch							
Afternoon Snack							

Food	Sunday	Monday	Tuesday	Wednesday	Thursday	Friday	Saturday
Dinner							
Evening Snack							
Drinks							

Suspected reactions or patterns: ____________________

Food/drink before migraine symptoms: ____________________

Patterns or combinations that stood out: ____________________

Comparison with migraine calendar: ____________________

Week 4 Food & Drink Journal

Date / /20______

Food	Sunday	Monday	Tuesday	Wednesday	Thursday	Friday	Saturday
Breakfast							
Morning Snack							
Lunch							
Afternoon Snack							

Food	Sunday	Monday	Tuesday	Wednesday	Thursday	Friday	Saturday
Dinner							
Evening Snack							
Drinks							

Suspected reactions or patterns: ______________________________

Food/drink before migraine symptoms: ______________________________

Patterns or combinations that stood out: ______________________________

Comparison with migraine calendar: ______________________________

Month 2

Monthly Migraine Trackers

Month 2: ____________________ 20______

	Day 1	2	3	4	5	6	7	8	9	10	11	12	13	14	15	16	17	18	19	20	21	22	23	24	25	26	27	28	29	30	31
Severity																															
Treatment																															
Effect																															
Sleep Issues																															
Stress/Emotion																															
Food/Diet																															
Menstrual																															
Weather																															
Exercise																															

Migraine Days ______ Medication Days_______ Avg Severity _____

Days with: Stress_____ Food/diet _______________ Menstrual _______

MEDICATION CODES

6. ______________________________

7. ______________________________

8. ______________________________

9. ______________________________

10. ______________________________

KEY

- Severity Scale: 0 = no pain, 5 = severe
- Treatment Effect: 1 = no effect 5 = complete relief
- Sleep Issues: 1 = Slept well 5 = Broken sleep / poor quality
- Stress/Emotion: 1 = calm/stable 5 = very high/extreme
- Food/Diet: ate food commonly linked with migraine
- Weather: 1 = stable 5 = extreme. Optional: S storm, P pressure change, H heat/heatwave, C cold/sudden drop, W wind
- Exercise: 1 = no activity, 5 = very intense exercise

Monthly Food & Hydration Tracker

Month 2: ________________ 20______

Check if you consumed common trigger foods. Track water intake and note any suspected reactions. If you do not know if you have any food triggers, track your daily food consumption using the pages at the end of this set. Track the 8oz water cups per day on the last row.

Day	1	2	3	4	5	6	7	8	9	10	11	12	13	14	15	16	17	18	19	20	21	22	23	24	25	26	27	28	29	30	31
Caffeine																															
Alcohol																															
Processed Food																															
Fermented Food																															
Dairy																															
Chocolate																															
Citrus																															
Water Cups																															

Suspected Reactions____

Monthly Sleep Tracker

Month 2: ____________________ 20______

Use the sleep quality scale to record your sleep hours and quality. Note any disruptions.

Day	1	2	3	4	5	6	7	8	9	10	11	12	13	14	15	16	17	18	19	20	21	22	23	24	25	26	27	28	29	30	31
Sleep Quality																															
Bedtime																															
Wake Time																															
Trouble falling asleep Y/N																															
# times awake																															
Meds/Supps																															
Naps																															

Sleep Quality Scale

6. Poor: Restless, multiple awakenings
7. Fair: Some tossing/turning, a few awakenings
8. Average: Generally restful with minor disruptions
9. Good: Solid sleep, woke feeling somewhat refreshed
10. Excellent: Deep sleep, woke feeling completely refreshed

Medications/Supplements Key

Example - Melatonin: M

Monthly Stress & Emotional Tracker

Month 2: ________________ 20_____

Each day, mark your stress level (1–5, with 5 being most intense), tick any emotions you felt, add an asterisk (*) if you had a migraine, and record stress relief using the codes below

Day	1	2	3	4	5	6	7	8	9	10	11	12	13	14	15	16	17	18	19	20	21	22	23	24	25	26	27	28	29	30	31
Stress level																															
Anxious																															
Sad																															
Angry																															
Worried																															
Calm																															
Happy																															
Tired																															
Overwhelmed																															
Stress Relief																															

Key For Stress Relief Activities

Deep breathing (D)
Walking (W)
Reading (R)
Bath/shower (B)
Meditation (M)
Exercise (E)
Socializing (S)
Music (C)
Other (O): ________________

Biggest stressors this month were: ________________________________

____

Stress relief that worked best and when was: ______________________

I noticed migraines most often when I felt: ______________________

Menstrual Cycle Tracker

Month 2: ____________ 20____

Many people with migraine notice changes around their menstrual cycle. Attacks are most likely to occur in the days just before and just after a period begins, sometimes called the menstrual migraine window. For some, migraines also appear with ovulation, spotting, or during heavier flow.

Tracking your cycle alongside migraine activity can help show patterns that may otherwise be hard to spot.

If you are perimenopausal or postmenopausal, you may find the monthly or episodic trackers more useful for noticing patterns.

Day	1	2	3	4	5	6	7	8	9	10	11	12	13	14	15	16	17	18	19	20	21	22	23	24	25	26	27	28	29	30	31
Period Day																															
Flow																															
Ovulation																															
Symptoms																															
Other																															

Start at Cycle Day 1 on the first day of bleeding and number forward until your next period begins. Tick or shade boxes for Period Days, Spotting, and Other Symptoms as needed. Use the Flow codes below to record daily flow.

Key For Symptoms

Migraine (*)	Tender breasts (T)
Headache (H)	Nausea / GI changes (N)
Cramps (C)	Sleep changes (S)
Bloating (B)	Hot flush/night sweat (X)
Fatigue/Tiredness (F)	Other ( ):
Mood changes (M)	

Note any hormonal treatments, or natural hormonal changes affecting your migraines. Even small shifts can sometimes change migraine patterns:

____

____

____

Monthly Medication & Supplement Tracker

Month 2: ________________ 20______

Write your medications and supplements in the key below (include dose). Each row is one medication/supplement. Tick on the days you take it. If you take more than once a day, add a tick for each dose. Use the notes section for side effects, missed doses, or anything unusual.

Meds/Supp	1	2	3	4	5	6	7	8	9	10	11	12	13	14	15	16	17	18	19	20	21	22	23	24	25	26	27	28	29	30	31

Key For Medications and Supplements

1. ____________________
2. ____________________
3. ____________________
4. ____________________
5. ____________________
6. ____________________
7. ____________________
8. ____________________
9. ____________________
10. ____________________

Notes

____

____

____

____

____

Monthly Tracker ______________________

Month: ______________ 20____

Track anything that is unique to you. Use the key and notes below to customize the tracker to suit.

	1	2	3	4	5	6	7	8	9	10	11	12	13	14	15	16	17	18	19	20	21	22	23	24	25	26	27	28	29	30	31

Key

Notes

Monthly Tracker ______________________ Month: ______________ 20____

Track anything that is unique to you. Use the key and notes below to customize the tracker to suit.

	1	2	3	4	5	6	7	8	9	10	11	12	13	14	15	16	17	18	19	20	21	22	23	24	25	26	27	28	29	30	31

Key

Notes

Monthly Tracker ____________________

Month: ______________ 20____

Track anything that is unique to you. Use the key and notes below to customize the tracker to suit.

	1	2	3	4	5	6	7	8	9	10	11	12	13	14	15	16	17	18	19	20	21	22	23	24	25	26	27	28	29	30	31

Key

Notes

Week 1 Food & Drink Journal

Date / /20______

Food	Sunday	Monday	Tuesday	Wednesday	Thursday	Friday	Saturday
Breakfast							
Morning Snack							
Lunch							
Afternoon Snack							

Food	Sunday	Monday	Tuesday	Wednesday	Thursday	Friday	Saturday
Dinner							
Evening Snack							
Drinks							

Suspected reactions or patterns: ______________________________

Food/drink before migraine symptoms: ______________________________

Patterns or combinations that stood out: ______________________________

Comparison with migraine calendar: ______________________________

Week 2 Food & Drink Journal

Date / /20______

Food	Sunday	Monday	Tuesday	Wednesday	Thursday	Friday	Saturday
Breakfast							
Morning Snack							
Lunch							
Afternoon Snack							

Food	Sunday	Monday	Tuesday	Wednesday	Thursday	Friday	Saturday
Dinner							
Evening Snack							
Drinks							

Suspected reactions or patterns: ______________________________

Food/drink before migraine symptoms: ______________________________

Patterns or combinations that stood out: ______________________________

Comparison with migraine calendar: ______________________________

Week 3 Food & Drink Journal

Date / /20______

Food	Sunday	Monday	Tuesday	Wednesday	Thursday	Friday	Saturday
Breakfast							
Morning Snack							
Lunch							
Afternoon Snack							

Food	Sunday	Monday	Tuesday	Wednesday	Thursday	Friday	Saturday
Dinner							
Evening Snack							
Drinks							

Suspected reactions or patterns: ______________________________

Food/drink before migraine symptoms: ______________________________

Patterns or combinations that stood out: ______________________________

Comparison with migraine calendar: ______________________________

Week 4 Food & Drink Journal

Date / /20_____

Food	Sunday	Monday	Tuesday	Wednesday	Thursday	Friday	Saturday
Breakfast							
Morning Snack							
Lunch							
Afternoon Snack							

Food	Sunday	Monday	Tuesday	Wednesday	Thursday	Friday	Saturday
Dinner							
Evening Snack							
Drinks							

Suspected reactions or patterns: ______________________________

Food/drink before migraine symptoms: ______________________________

Patterns or combinations that stood out: ______________________________

Comparison with migraine calendar: ______________________________

Month 3

Monthly Migraine Trackers

Month 3: ______________________20________

	Day 1	2	3	4	5	6	7	8	9	10	11	12	13	14	15	16	17	18	19	20	21	22	23	24	25	26	27	28	29	30	31
Severity																															
Treatment																															
Effect																															
Sleep Issues																															
Stress/Emotion																															
Food/Diet																															
Menstrual																															
Weather																															
Exercise																															

Migraine Days ________ Medication Days________ Avg Severity ______

Days with: Stress_____ Food/diet ______________ Menstrual _______

MEDICATION CODES

11. ____

12. ____

13. ____

14. ____

15. ____

KEY

- Severity Scale: 0 = no pain, 5 = severe
- Treatment Effect: 1 = no effect 5 = complete relief
- Sleep Issues: 1 = Slept well 5 = Broken sleep / poor quality
- Stress/Emotion: 1 = calm/stable 5 = very high/extreme
- Food/Diet: ate food commonly linked with migraine
- Weather: 1 = stable 5 = extreme. Optional: S storm, P pressure change, H heat/heatwave, C cold/sudden drop, W wind
- Exercise: 1 = no activity, 5 = very intense exercise

Monthly Food & Hydration Tracker

Month 3: ________________ 20______

Check if you consumed common trigger foods. Track water intake and note any suspected reactions. If you do not know if you have any food triggers, track your daily food consumption using the pages at the end of this set. Track the 8oz water cups per day on the last row.

Day	1	2	3	4	5	6	7	8	9	10	11	12	13	14	15	16	17	18	19	20	21	22	23	24	25	26	27	28	29	30	31
Caffeine																															
Alcohol																															
Processed Food																															
Fermented Food																															
Dairy																															
Chocolate																															
Citrus																															
Water Cups																															

Suspected Reactions____

____

____

____

____

Monthly Sleep Tracker

Month 3: ____________________ 20______

Use the sleep quality scale to record your sleep hours and quality. Note any disruptions.

Day	1	2	3	4	5	6	7	8	9	10	11	12	13	14	15	16	17	18	19	20	21	22	23	24	25	26	27	28	29	30	31
Sleep Quality																															
Bedtime																															
Wake Time																															
Trouble falling asleep Y/N																															
# times awake																															
Meds/Supps																															
Naps																															

Sleep Quality Scale

11. Poor: Restless, multiple awakenings
12. Fair: Some tossing/turning, a few awakenings
13. Average: Generally restful with minor disruptions
14. Good: Solid sleep, woke feeling somewhat refreshed
15. Excellent: Deep sleep, woke feeling completely refreshed

Medications/Supplements Key

Example - Melatonin: M

Monthly Stress & Emotional Tracker

Month 3: ______________ 20_____

Each day, mark your stress level (1–5, with 5 being most intense), tick any emotions you felt, add an asterisk (*) if you had a migraine, and record stress relief using the codes below

Day	1	2	3	4	5	6	7	8	9	10	11	12	13	14	15	16	17	18	19	20	21	22	23	24	25	26	27	28	29	30	31
Stress level																															
Anxious																															
Sad																															
Angry																															
Worried																															
Calm																															
Happy																															
Tired																															
Overwhelmed																															
Stress Relief																															

Key For Stress Relief Activities

Deep breathing (D)	Exercise (E)
Walking (W)	Socializing (S)
Reading (R)	Music (C)
Bath/shower (B)	Other (O): ______________
Meditation (M)	

Biggest stressors this month were: ______________

____

Stress relief that worked best and when was: ______________

I noticed migraines most often when I felt: ______________

Menstrual Cycle Tracker

Month 3: ____________________ 20______

Many people with migraine notice changes around their menstrual cycle. Attacks are most likely to occur in the days just before and just after a period begins, sometimes called the menstrual migraine window. For some, migraines also appear with ovulation, spotting, or during heavier flow.

Tracking your cycle alongside migraine activity can help show patterns that may otherwise be hard to spot.

If you are perimenopausal or postmenopausal, you may find the monthly or episodic trackers more useful for noticing patterns.

Day	1	2	3	4	5	6	7	8	9	10	11	12	13	14	15	16	17	18	19	20	21	22	23	24	25	26	27	28	29	30	31
Period Day																															
Flow																															
Ovulation																															
Symptoms																															
Other																															

Start at Cycle Day 1 on the first day of bleeding and number forward until your next period begins. Tick or shade boxes for Period Days, Spotting, and Other Symptoms as needed. Use the Flow codes below to record daily flow.

Key For Symptoms

Migraine (*)	Tender breasts (T)
Headache (H)	Nausea / GI changes (N)
Cramps (C)	Sleep changes (S)
Bloating (B)	Hot flush/night sweat (X)
Fatigue/Tiredness (F)	Other ( ):
Mood changes (M)	

Note any hormonal treatments, or natural hormonal changes affecting your migraines. Even small shifts can sometimes change migraine patterns:

____

____

____

Monthly Medication & Supplement Tracker

Month 2: ________________ 20______

Write your medications and supplements in the key below (include dose). Each row is one medication/supplement. Tick on the days you take it. If you take more than once a day, add a tick for each dose. Use the notes section for side effects, missed doses, or anything unusual.

Meds/Supp	1	2	3	4	5	6	7	8	9	10	11	12	13	14	15	16	17	18	19	20	21	22	23	24	25	26	27	28	29	30	31

Key For Medications and Supplements

1. ____________________
2. ____________________
3. ____________________
4. ____________________
5. ____________________
6. ____________________
7. ____________________
8. ____________________
9. ____________________
10. ____________________

Notes

____

____

____

____

____

Monthly Tracker ______________________

Month: ______________ 20_____

Track anything that is unique to you. Use the key and notes below to customize the tracker to suit.

	1	2	3	4	5	6	7	8	9	10	11	12	13	14	15	16	17	18	19	20	21	22	23	24	25	26	27	28	29	30	31

Key

Notes

Monthly Tracker ______________________

Month: ________________ 20_____

Track anything that is unique to you. Use the key and notes below to customize the tracker to suit.

	1	2	3	4	5	6	7	8	9	10	11	12	13	14	15	16	17	18	19	20	21	22	23	24	25	26	27	28	29	30	31

Key

Notes

Monthly Tracker ____________________

Month: ______________ 20_____

Track anything that is unique to you. Use the key and notes below to customize the tracker to suit.

	1	2	3	4	5	6	7	8	9	10	11	12	13	14	15	16	17	18	19	20	21	22	23	24	25	26	27	28	29	30	31

Key

Notes

Week 1 Food & Drink Journal

Date / /20______

Food	Sunday	Monday	Tuesday	Wednesday	Thursday	Friday	Saturday
Breakfast							
Morning Snack							
Lunch							
Afternoon Snack							

Food	Sunday	Monday	Tuesday	Wednesday	Thursday	Friday	Saturday
Dinner							
Evening Snack							
Drinks							

Suspected reactions or patterns: ____________________

Food/drink before migraine symptoms: ____________________

Patterns or combinations that stood out: ____________________

Comparison with migraine calendar: ____________________

Week 2 Food & Drink Journal

Date / /20______

Food	Sunday	Monday	Tuesday	Wednesday	Thursday	Friday	Saturday
Breakfast							
Morning Snack							
Lunch							
Afternoon Snack							

Food	Sunday	Monday	Tuesday	Wednesday	Thursday	Friday	Saturday
Dinner							
Evening Snack							
Drinks							

Suspected reactions or patterns: ______________________________

Food/drink before migraine symptoms: ______________________________

Patterns or combinations that stood out: ______________________________

Comparison with migraine calendar: ______________________________

Week 3 Food & Drink Journal

Date / /20______

Food	Sunday	Monday	Tuesday	Wednesday	Thursday	Friday	Saturday
Breakfast							
Morning Snack							
Lunch							
Afternoon Snack							

Food	Sunday	Monday	Tuesday	Wednesday	Thursday	Friday	Saturday
Dinner							
Evening Snack							
Drinks							

Suspected reactions or patterns: ____________________

Food/drink before migraine symptoms: ____________________

Patterns or combinations that stood out: ____________________

Comparison with migraine calendar: ____________________

Week 4 Food & Drink Journal

Date / /20______

Food	Sunday	Monday	Tuesday	Wednesday	Thursday	Friday	Saturday
Breakfast							
Morning Snack							
Lunch							
Afternoon Snack							

Food	Sunday	Monday	Tuesday	Wednesday	Thursday	Friday	Saturday
Dinner							
Evening Snack							
Drinks							

Suspected reactions or patterns: ____________________

Food/drink before migraine symptoms: ____________________

Patterns or combinations that stood out: ____________________

Comparison with migraine calendar: ____________________

Section 2 Episode Trackers

While the monthly and focused trackers in Section 1 give you the broader picture, some attacks call for more detail. The episode trackers in this section provide space to record individual migraines, especially those that were severe, unusual, or didn't respond well to treatment.

Each log guides you through the full course of an attack, from early warning signs and suspected triggers to treatment strategies, recovery, and impact on daily activities. Completing a log soon after an attack makes it easier to capture details you might otherwise forget.

You do not need to fill in every box for these pages to be valuable. Even partial notes can show patterns over time, highlight effective strategies, and provide clear information to share with your healthcare provider.

Over time, these detailed records combine with the monthly and focused trackers to give you both a wide view and a close-up picture of your migraine experience.

Migraine Episode Tracker

Complete as much of this log as you can. Even partial notes are valuable. Use for migraines that were severe, unusual, or didn't respond well to treatment.

Episode #	Date Started: / /20	Time

ONSET AND EARLY SYMPTOMS

Prodrome

☐ Mood changes ☐ Food cravings ☐ Yawning ☐ Thirst

☐ Frequent urination ☐ Fatigue ☐ Neck stiffness

☐ Concentration ☐ Smell sensitive ☐ Other: ____________________

Aura

☐ Visual changes ☐ Numbness/tingling ☐ Speech difficulty

☐ Weakness ☐ Dizziness ☐ Other: ____________________

HEADACHE PHASE

Pain location

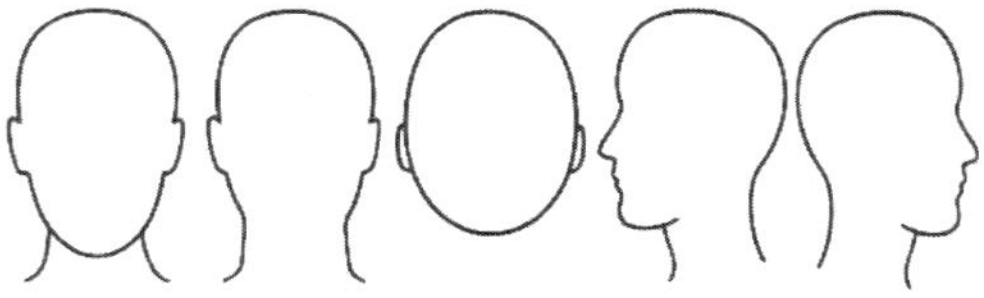

FRONT BACK TOP LEFT RIGHT

Pain quality:

☐ Throbbing ☐ Pressure

☐ Stabbing ☐ Burning

☐ Tight ☐ Other:

Intensity: 0 1 2 3 4 5

Other symptoms:

☐ Nausea ☐ Vomiting ☐ Dizziness ☐ Fatigue

☐ Confusion ☐ Neck pain ☐ Vision changes ☐ Anxiety

☐ Light sensitivity ☐ Sound sensitivity ☐ Smell sensitivity ☐ Skin sensitivity

☐ Other:

TRIGGERS

Tick any factors you believe/suspect contributed to this episode, even if you also tracked them in your monthly log.

☐ Stress/emotion ☐ Food/drink ☐ Weather/environment

☐ Exercise/activity ☐ Hormonal ☐ Screen time

☐ Other:

RELIEF STRATEGIES & MEDICATIONS USED

List medications and non-medication strategies (rest, dark room, cold/heat packs, hydration, sleep, relaxation techniques, etc.

Time (approx.)	Medication/ Strategy	Effective? (1 no relief-5 complete)	Side Effects	Rebound Y/N

RESOLUTION AND POSTDROME

End Date: / / Time ____________ Total Duration ____________

How it ended

☐ Gradual ☐ Sudden ☐ Other

Postdrome Symptoms

☐ Fatigue ☐ Confusion ☐ Mood changes

☐ Head pain with movement ☐ Light/sound sensitivity

☐ Other:

Impact:

Missed activities, work, social plans?

NOTES: Unusual symptoms, suspected new triggers, reflections, etc.

____

____

____

Migraine Episode Tracker

Complete as much of this log as you can. Even partial notes are valuable. Use for migraines that were severe, unusual, or didn't respond well to treatment.

Episode # Date Started: / /20 Time

ONSET AND EARLY SYMPTOMS

Prodrome

☐ Mood changes ☐ Food cravings ☐ Yawning ☐ Thirst

☐ Frequent urination ☐ Fatigue ☐ Neck stiffness

☐ Concentration ☐ Smell sensitive ☐ Other: ____________________

Aura

☐ Visual changes ☐ Numbness/tingling ☐ Speech difficulty

☐ Weakness ☐ Dizziness ☐ Other: ____________________

HEADACHE PHASE

Pain location

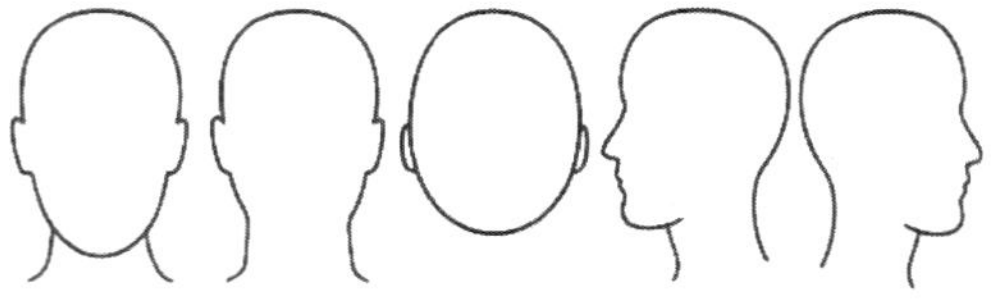

FRONT BACK TOP LEFT RIGHT

Pain quality:

☐ Throbbing ☐ Pressure

☐ Stabbing ☐ Burning

☐ Tight ☐ Other:

Intensity: 0 1 2 3 4 5

Other symptoms:

☐ Nausea ☐ Vomiting ☐ Dizziness ☐ Fatigue

☐ Confusion ☐ Neck pain ☐ Vision changes ☐ Anxiety

☐ Light sensitivity ☐ Sound sensitivity ☐ Smell sensitivity ☐ Skin sensitivity

☐ Other:

TRIGGERS

Tick any factors you believe/suspect contributed to this episode, even if you also tracked them in your monthly log.

☐ Stress/emotion ☐ Food/drink ☐ Weather/environment

☐ Exercise/activity ☐ Hormonal ☐ Screen time

☐ Other:

RELIEF STRATEGIES & MEDICATIONS USED

List medications and non-medication strategies (rest, dark room, cold/heat packs, hydration, sleep, relaxation techniques, etc.

Time (approx.)	Medication/ Strategy	Effective? (1 no relief-5 complete)	Side Effects	Rebound Y/N

RESOLUTION AND POSTDROME

End Date: / / Time ____________ Total Duration ____________

How it ended

☐ Gradual ☐ Sudden ☐ Other

Postdrome Symptoms

☐ Fatigue ☐ Confusion ☐ Mood changes

☐ Head pain with movement ☐ Light/sound sensitivity

☐ Other:

Impact:

Missed activities, work, social plans?

NOTES: Unusual symptoms, suspected new triggers, reflections, etc.

____

____

____

Migraine Episode Tracker

Complete as much of this log as you can. Even partial notes are valuable. Use for migraines that were severe, unusual, or didn't respond well to treatment.

Episode # Date Started: / /20 Time

ONSET AND EARLY SYMPTOMS

Prodrome

☐ Mood changes ☐ Food cravings ☐ Yawning ☐ Thirst

☐ Frequent urination ☐ Fatigue ☐ Neck stiffness

☐ Concentration ☐ Smell sensitive ☐ Other: ____________________

Aura

☐ Visual changes ☐ Numbness/tingling ☐ Speech difficulty

☐ Weakness ☐ Dizziness ☐ Other: ____________________

HEADACHE PHASE

Pain location

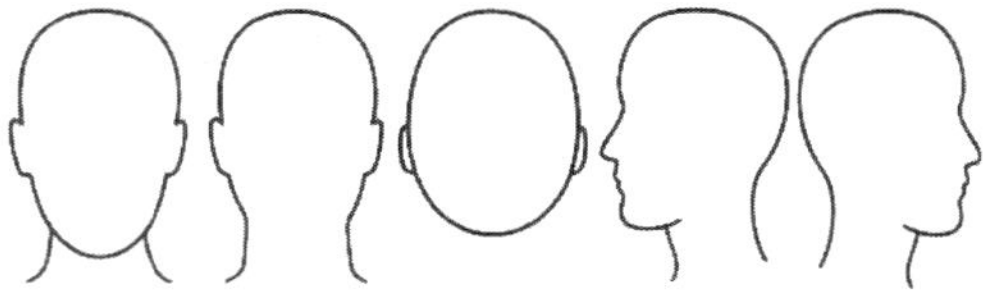

FRONT BACK TOP LEFT RIGHT

Pain quality:

☐ Throbbing ☐ Pressure

☐ Stabbing ☐ Burning

☐ Tight ☐ Other:

Intensity: 0 1 2 3 4 5

Other symptoms:

☐ Nausea ☐ Vomiting ☐ Dizziness ☐ Fatigue

☐ Confusion ☐ Neck pain ☐ Vision changes ☐ Anxiety

☐ Light sensitivity ☐ Sound sensitivity ☐ Smell sensitivity ☐ Skin sensitivity

☐ Other:

TRIGGERS

Tick any factors you believe/suspect contributed to this episode, even if you also tracked them in your monthly log.

☐ Stress/emotion ☐ Food/drink ☐ Weather/environment

☐ Exercise/activity ☐ Hormonal ☐ Screen time

☐ Other:

RELIEF STRATEGIES & MEDICATIONS USED

List medications and non-medication strategies (rest, dark room, cold/heat packs, hydration, sleep, relaxation techniques, etc.

Time (approx.)	Medication/ Strategy	Effective? (1 no relief-5 complete)	Side Effects	Rebound Y/N

RESOLUTION AND POSTDROME

End Date: / / Time ____________ Total Duration ____________

How it ended

☐ Gradual ☐ Sudden ☐ Other

Postdrome Symptoms

☐ Fatigue ☐ Confusion ☐ Mood changes

☐ Head pain with movement ☐ Light/sound sensitivity

☐ Other:

Impact:

Missed activities, work, social plans?

NOTES: Unusual symptoms, suspected new triggers, reflections, etc.

____

____

____

Migraine Episode Tracker

Complete as much of this log as you can. Even partial notes are valuable. Use for migraines that were severe, unusual, or didn't respond well to treatment.

Episode # Date Started: / /20 Time

ONSET AND EARLY SYMPTOMS

Prodrome

☐ Mood changes ☐ Food cravings ☐ Yawning ☐ Thirst

☐ Frequent urination ☐ Fatigue ☐ Neck stiffness

☐ Concentration ☐ Smell sensitive ☐ Other: ____________________

Aura

☐ Visual changes ☐ Numbness/tingling ☐ Speech difficulty

☐ Weakness ☐ Dizziness ☐ Other: ____________________

HEADACHE PHASE

Pain location

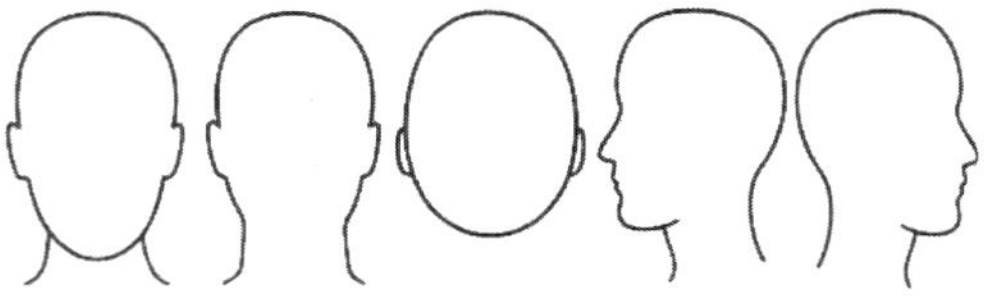

FRONT BACK TOP LEFT RIGHT

Pain quality:

☐ Throbbing ☐ Pressure

☐ Stabbing ☐ Burning

☐ Tight ☐ Other:

Intensity: 0 1 2 3 4 5

Other symptoms:

☐ Nausea ☐ Vomiting ☐ Dizziness ☐ Fatigue

☐ Confusion ☐ Neck pain ☐ Vision changes ☐ Anxiety

☐ Light sensitivity ☐ Sound sensitivity ☐ Smell sensitivity ☐ Skin sensitivity

☐ Other:

TRIGGERS

Tick any factors you believe/suspect contributed to this episode, even if you also tracked them in your monthly log.

☐ Stress/emotion ☐ Food/drink ☐ Weather/environment

☐ Exercise/activity ☐ Hormonal ☐ Screen time

☐ Other:

RELIEF STRATEGIES & MEDICATIONS USED

List medications and non-medication strategies (rest, dark room, cold/heat packs, hydration, sleep, relaxation techniques, etc.

Time (approx.)	Medication/ Strategy	Effective? (1 no relief-5 complete)	Side Effects	Rebound Y/N

RESOLUTION AND POSTDROME

End Date: / / Time ____________ Total Duration ____________

How it ended

☐ Gradual ☐ Sudden ☐ Other

Postdrome Symptoms

☐ Fatigue ☐ Confusion ☐ Mood changes

☐ Head pain with movement ☐ Light/sound sensitivity

☐ Other:

Impact:

Missed activities, work, social plans?

NOTES: Unusual symptoms, suspected new triggers, reflections, etc.

____

____

____

Migraine Episode Tracker

Complete as much of this log as you can. Even partial notes are valuable. Use for migraines that were severe, unusual, or didn't respond well to treatment.

Episode # Date Started: / /20 Time

ONSET AND EARLY SYMPTOMS

Prodrome

☐ Mood changes ☐ Food cravings ☐ Yawning ☐ Thirst

☐ Frequent urination ☐ Fatigue ☐ Neck stiffness

☐ Concentration ☐ Smell sensitive ☐ Other: ____________________

Aura

☐ Visual changes ☐ Numbness/tingling ☐ Speech difficulty

☐ Weakness ☐ Dizziness ☐ Other: ____________________

HEADACHE PHASE

Pain location

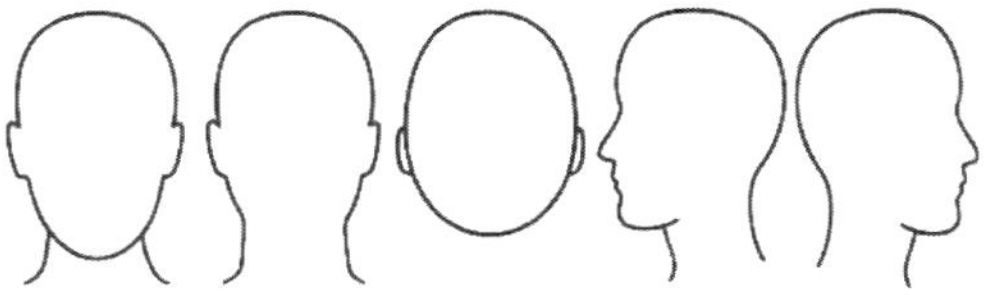

FRONT BACK TOP LEFT RIGHT

Pain quality:

☐ Throbbing ☐ Pressure

☐ Stabbing ☐ Burning

☐ Tight ☐ Other:

Intensity: 0 1 2 3 4 5

Other symptoms:

☐ Nausea ☐ Vomiting ☐ Dizziness ☐ Fatigue

☐ Confusion ☐ Neck pain ☐ Vision changes ☐ Anxiety

☐ Light sensitivity ☐ Sound sensitivity ☐ Smell sensitivity ☐ Skin sensitivity

☐ Other:

TRIGGERS

Tick any factors you believe/suspect contributed to this episode, even if you also tracked them in your monthly log.

☐ Stress/emotion ☐ Food/drink ☐ Weather/environment

☐ Exercise/activity ☐ Hormonal ☐ Screen time

☐ Other:

RELIEF STRATEGIES & MEDICATIONS USED

List medications and non-medication strategies (rest, dark room, cold/heat packs, hydration, sleep, relaxation techniques, etc.

Time (approx.)	Medication/ Strategy	Effective? (1 no relief-5 complete)	Side Effects	Rebound Y/N

RESOLUTION AND POSTDROME

End Date: / / Time ____________ Total Duration ____________

How it ended

☐ Gradual ☐ Sudden ☐ Other

Postdrome Symptoms

☐ Fatigue ☐ Confusion ☐ Mood changes

☐ Head pain with movement ☐ Light/sound sensitivity

☐ Other:

Impact:

Missed activities, work, social plans?

NOTES: Unusual symptoms, suspected new triggers, reflections, etc.

___

___

___

Migraine Episode Tracker

Complete as much of this log as you can. Even partial notes are valuable. Use for migraines that were severe, unusual, or didn't respond well to treatment.

Episode #   Date Started: /   /20   Time

ONSET AND EARLY SYMPTOMS

Prodrome

☐ Mood changes ☐ Food cravings ☐ Yawning ☐ Thirst

☐ Frequent urination ☐ Fatigue ☐ Neck stiffness

☐ Concentration ☐ Smell sensitive ☐ Other: ____________________

Aura

☐ Visual changes ☐ Numbness/tingling ☐ Speech difficulty

☐ Weakness ☐ Dizziness ☐ Other: ____________________

HEADACHE PHASE

Pain location

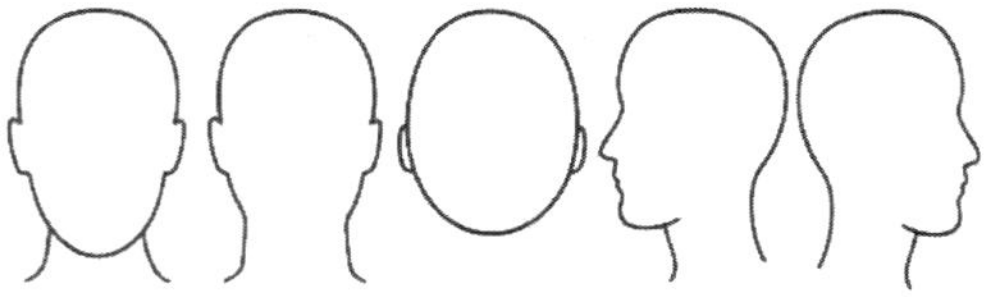

FRONT BACK TOP LEFT RIGHT

Pain quality:

☐ Throbbing ☐ Pressure

☐ Stabbing ☐ Burning

☐ Tight ☐ Other:

Intensity: 0 1 2 3 4 5

Other symptoms:

☐ Nausea ☐ Vomiting ☐ Dizziness ☐ Fatigue

☐ Confusion ☐ Neck pain ☐ Vision changes ☐ Anxiety

☐ Light sensitivity ☐ Sound sensitivity ☐ Smell sensitivity ☐ Skin sensitivity

☐ Other:

TRIGGERS

Tick any factors you believe/suspect contributed to this episode, even if you also tracked them in your monthly log.

☐ Stress/emotion ☐ Food/drink ☐ Weather/environment

☐ Exercise/activity ☐ Hormonal ☐ Screen time

☐ Other:

RELIEF STRATEGIES & MEDICATIONS USED

List medications and non-medication strategies (rest, dark room, cold/heat packs, hydration, sleep, relaxation techniques, etc.

Time (approx.)	Medication/ Strategy	Effective? (1 no relief-5 complete)	Side Effects	Rebound Y/N

RESOLUTION AND POSTDROME

End Date: / / Time ____________ Total Duration ____________

How it ended

☐ Gradual ☐ Sudden ☐ Other

Postdrome Symptoms

☐ Fatigue ☐ Confusion ☐ Mood changes

☐ Head pain with movement ☐ Light/sound sensitivity

☐ Other:

Impact:

Missed activities, work, social plans?

NOTES: Unusual symptoms, suspected new triggers, reflections, etc.

____

____

____

Migraine Episode Tracker

Complete as much of this log as you can. Even partial notes are valuable. Use for migraines that were severe, unusual, or didn't respond well to treatment.

Episode # Date Started: / /20 Time

ONSET AND EARLY SYMPTOMS

Prodrome

☐ Mood changes ☐ Food cravings ☐ Yawning ☐ Thirst

☐ Frequent urination ☐ Fatigue ☐ Neck stiffness

☐ Concentration ☐ Smell sensitive ☐ Other: ____________________

Aura

☐ Visual changes ☐ Numbness/tingling ☐ Speech difficulty

☐ Weakness ☐ Dizziness ☐ Other: ____________________

HEADACHE PHASE

Pain location

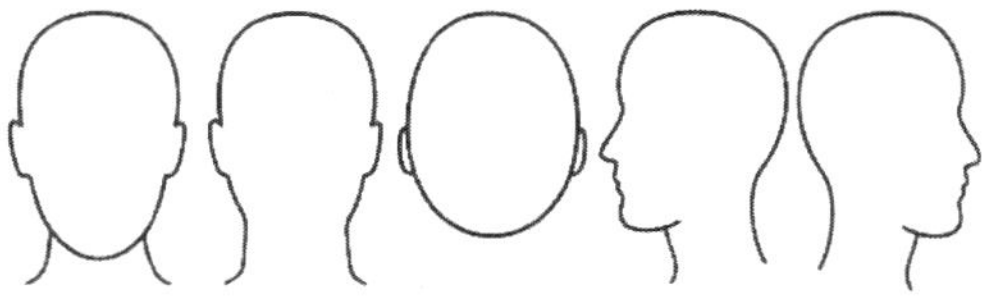

FRONT BACK TOP LEFT RIGHT

Pain quality:

☐ Throbbing ☐ Pressure

☐ Stabbing ☐ Burning

☐ Tight ☐ Other:

Intensity: 0 1 2 3 4 5

Other symptoms:

☐ Nausea ☐ Vomiting ☐ Dizziness ☐ Fatigue

☐ Confusion ☐ Neck pain ☐ Vision changes ☐ Anxiety

☐ Light sensitivity ☐ Sound sensitivity ☐ Smell sensitivity ☐ Skin sensitivity

☐ Other:

TRIGGERS

Tick any factors you believe/suspect contributed to this episode, even if you also tracked them in your monthly log.

☐ Stress/emotion ☐ Food/drink ☐ Weather/environment

☐ Exercise/activity ☐ Hormonal ☐ Screen time

☐ Other:

RELIEF STRATEGIES & MEDICATIONS USED

List medications and non-medication strategies (rest, dark room, cold/heat packs, hydration, sleep, relaxation techniques, etc.

Time (approx.)	Medication/ Strategy	Effective? (1 no relief-5 complete)	Side Effects	Rebound Y/N

RESOLUTION AND POSTDROME

End Date: / / Time ____________ Total Duration ____________

How it ended

☐ Gradual ☐ Sudden ☐ Other

Postdrome Symptoms

☐ Fatigue ☐ Confusion ☐ Mood changes

☐ Head pain with movement ☐ Light/sound sensitivity

☐ Other:

Impact:

Missed activities, work, social plans?

NOTES: Unusual symptoms, suspected new triggers, reflections, etc.

____

____

____

Migraine Episode Tracker

Complete as much of this log as you can. Even partial notes are valuable. Use for migraines that were severe, unusual, or didn't respond well to treatment.

Episode # Date Started: / /20 Time

ONSET AND EARLY SYMPTOMS

Prodrome

☐ Mood changes ☐ Food cravings ☐ Yawning ☐ Thirst
☐ Frequent urination ☐ Fatigue ☐ Neck stiffness
☐ Concentration ☐ Smell sensitive ☐ Other: ____________________

Aura

☐ Visual changes ☐ Numbness/tingling ☐ Speech difficulty
☐ Weakness ☐ Dizziness ☐ Other: ____________________

HEADACHE PHASE

Pain location

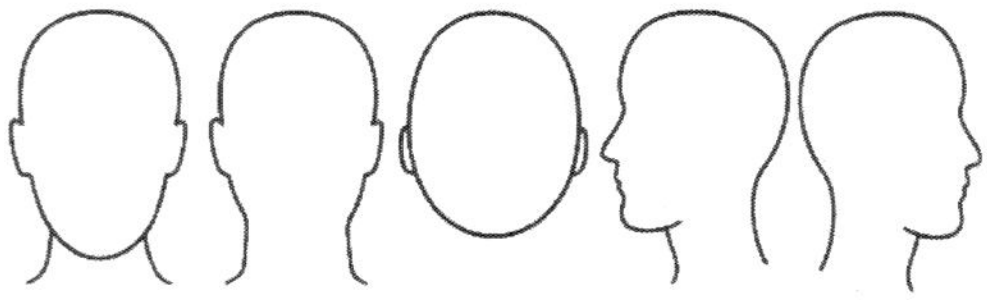

FRONT BACK TOP LEFT RIGHT

Pain quality:

☐ Throbbing ☐ Pressure
☐ Stabbing ☐ Burning
☐ Tight ☐ Other:

Intensity: 0 1 2 3 4 5

Other symptoms:

☐ Nausea ☐ Vomiting ☐ Dizziness ☐ Fatigue
☐ Confusion ☐ Neck pain ☐ Vision changes ☐ Anxiety
☐ Light sensitivity ☐ Sound sensitivity ☐ Smell sensitivity ☐ Skin sensitivity
☐ Other:

TRIGGERS

Tick any factors you believe/suspect contributed to this episode, even if you also tracked them in your monthly log.

☐ Stress/emotion ☐ Food/drink ☐ Weather/environment
☐ Exercise/activity ☐ Hormonal ☐ Screen time
☐ Other:

RELIEF STRATEGIES & MEDICATIONS USED

List medications and non-medication strategies (rest, dark room, cold/heat packs, hydration, sleep, relaxation techniques, etc.

Time (approx.)	Medication/ Strategy	Effective? (1 no relief-5 complete)	Side Effects	Rebound Y/N

RESOLUTION AND POSTDROME

End Date: / / Time ____________ Total Duration ____________

How it ended

☐ Gradual ☐ Sudden ☐ Other

Postdrome Symptoms

☐ Fatigue ☐ Confusion ☐ Mood changes

☐ Head pain with movement ☐ Light/sound sensitivity

☐ Other:

Impact:

Missed activities, work, social plans?

NOTES: Unusual symptoms, suspected new triggers, reflections, etc.

____

____

____

Migraine Episode Tracker

Complete as much of this log as you can. Even partial notes are valuable. Use for migraines that were severe, unusual, or didn't respond well to treatment.

Episode # Date Started: / /20 Time

ONSET AND EARLY SYMPTOMS

Prodrome

☐ Mood changes ☐ Food cravings ☐ Yawning ☐ Thirst

☐ Frequent urination ☐ Fatigue ☐ Neck stiffness

☐ Concentration ☐ Smell sensitive ☐ Other: ____________________

Aura

☐ Visual changes ☐ Numbness/tingling ☐ Speech difficulty

☐ Weakness ☐ Dizziness ☐ Other: ____________________

HEADACHE PHASE

Pain location

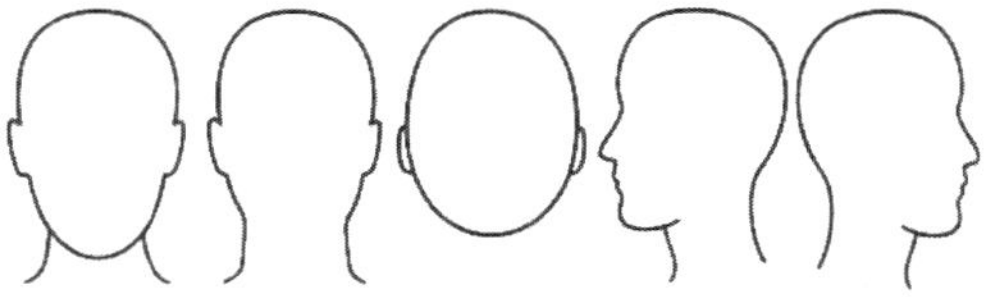

Pain quality:

☐ Throbbing ☐ Pressure

☐ Stabbing ☐ Burning

☐ Tight ☐ Other:

Intensity: 0 1 2 3 4 5

Other symptoms:

☐ Nausea ☐ Vomiting ☐ Dizziness ☐ Fatigue

☐ Confusion ☐ Neck pain ☐ Vision changes ☐ Anxiety

☐ Light sensitivity ☐ Sound sensitivity ☐ Smell sensitivity ☐ Skin sensitivity

☐ Other:

TRIGGERS

Tick any factors you believe/suspect contributed to this episode, even if you also tracked them in your monthly log.

☐ Stress/emotion ☐ Food/drink ☐ Weather/environment

☐ Exercise/activity ☐ Hormonal ☐ Screen time

☐ Other:

RELIEF STRATEGIES & MEDICATIONS USED

List medications and non-medication strategies (rest, dark room, cold/heat packs, hydration, sleep, relaxation techniques, etc.

Time (approx.)	Medication/ Strategy	Effective? (1 no relief-5 complete)	Side Effects	Rebound Y/N

RESOLUTION AND POSTDROME

End Date: / / Time ___________ Total Duration ___________

How it ended

☐ Gradual ☐ Sudden ☐ Other

Postdrome Symptoms

☐ Fatigue ☐ Confusion ☐ Mood changes

☐ Head pain with movement ☐ Light/sound sensitivity

☐ Other:

Impact:

Missed activities, work, social plans?

NOTES: Unusual symptoms, suspected new triggers, reflections, etc.

___

___

___

Migraine Episode Tracker

Complete as much of this log as you can. Even partial notes are valuable. Use for migraines that were severe, unusual, or didn't respond well to treatment.

Episode #	Date Started: / /20	Time

ONSET AND EARLY SYMPTOMS

Prodrome

☐ Mood changes ☐ Food cravings ☐ Yawning ☐ Thirst

☐ Frequent urination ☐ Fatigue ☐ Neck stiffness

☐ Concentration ☐ Smell sensitive ☐ Other: ____________________

Aura

☐ Visual changes ☐ Numbness/tingling ☐ Speech difficulty

☐ Weakness ☐ Dizziness ☐ Other: ____________________

HEADACHE PHASE

Pain location

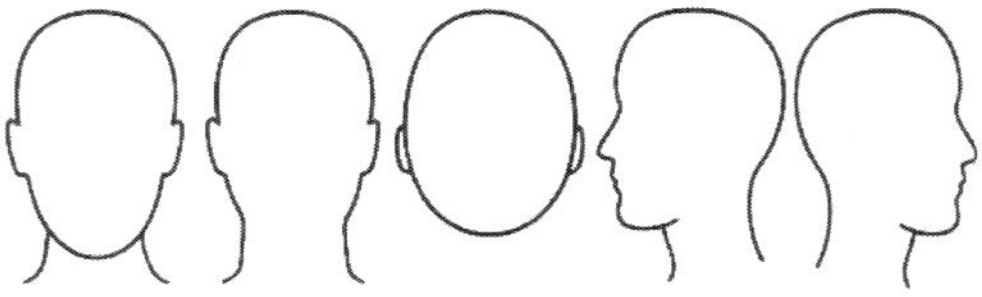

FRONT BACK TOP LEFT RIGHT

Pain quality:

☐ Throbbing ☐ Pressure

☐ Stabbing ☐ Burning

☐ Tight ☐ Other:

Intensity: 0 1 2 3 4 5

Other symptoms:

☐ Nausea ☐ Vomiting ☐ Dizziness ☐ Fatigue

☐ Confusion ☐ Neck pain ☐ Vision changes ☐ Anxiety

☐ Light sensitivity ☐ Sound sensitivity ☐ Smell sensitivity ☐ Skin sensitivity

☐ Other:

TRIGGERS

Tick any factors you believe/suspect contributed to this episode, even if you also tracked them in your monthly log.

☐ Stress/emotion ☐ Food/drink ☐ Weather/environment

☐ Exercise/activity ☐ Hormonal ☐ Screen time

☐ Other:

RELIEF STRATEGIES & MEDICATIONS USED

List medications and non-medication strategies (rest, dark room, cold/heat packs, hydration, sleep, relaxation techniques, etc.

Time (approx.)	Medication/ Strategy	Effective? (1 no relief-5 complete)	Side Effects	Rebound Y/N

RESOLUTION AND POSTDROME

End Date: / / Time ____________ Total Duration ____________

How it ended

☐ Gradual ☐ Sudden ☐ Other

Postdrome Symptoms

☐ Fatigue ☐ Confusion ☐ Mood changes

☐ Head pain with movement ☐ Light/sound sensitivity

☐ Other:

Impact:

Missed activities, work, social plans?

NOTES: Unusual symptoms, suspected new triggers, reflections, etc.

____

____

____

Migraine Episode Tracker

Complete as much of this log as you can. Even partial notes are valuable. Use for migraines that were severe, unusual, or didn't respond well to treatment.

Episode #   Date Started: /   /20   Time

ONSET AND EARLY SYMPTOMS

Prodrome

☐ Mood changes ☐ Food cravings ☐ Yawning ☐ Thirst

☐ Frequent urination ☐ Fatigue ☐ Neck stiffness

☐ Concentration ☐ Smell sensitive ☐ Other: ____________________

Aura

☐ Visual changes ☐ Numbness/tingling ☐ Speech difficulty

☐ Weakness ☐ Dizziness ☐ Other: ____________________

HEADACHE PHASE

Pain location

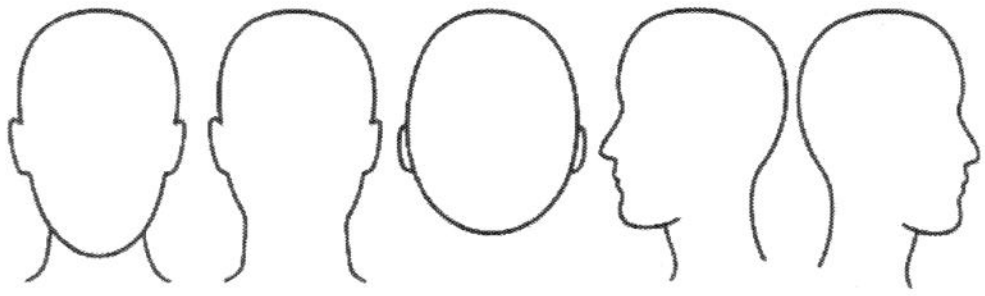

Pain quality:

☐ Throbbing ☐ Pressure

☐ Stabbing ☐ Burning

☐ Tight ☐ Other:

Intensity: 0 1 2 3 4 5

Other symptoms:

☐ Nausea ☐ Vomiting ☐ Dizziness ☐ Fatigue

☐ Confusion ☐ Neck pain ☐ Vision changes ☐ Anxiety

☐ Light sensitivity ☐ Sound sensitivity ☐ Smell sensitivity ☐ Skin sensitivity

☐ Other:

TRIGGERS

Tick any factors you believe/suspect contributed to this episode, even if you also tracked them in your monthly log.

☐ Stress/emotion ☐ Food/drink ☐ Weather/environment

☐ Exercise/activity ☐ Hormonal ☐ Screen time

☐ Other:

RELIEF STRATEGIES & MEDICATIONS USED

List medications and non-medication strategies (rest, dark room, cold/heat packs, hydration, sleep, relaxation techniques, etc.

Time (approx.)	Medication/ Strategy	Effective? (1 no relief-5 complete)	Side Effects	Rebound Y/N

RESOLUTION AND POSTDROME

End Date: / / Time ____________ Total Duration ____________

How it ended

☐ Gradual ☐ Sudden ☐ Other

Postdrome Symptoms

☐ Fatigue ☐ Confusion ☐ Mood changes

☐ Head pain with movement ☐ Light/sound sensitivity

☐ Other:

Impact:

Missed activities, work, social plans?

NOTES: Unusual symptoms, suspected new triggers, reflections, etc.

____

____

____

Migraine Episode Tracker

Complete as much of this log as you can. Even partial notes are valuable. Use for migraines that were severe, unusual, or didn't respond well to treatment.

Episode # Date Started: / /20 Time

ONSET AND EARLY SYMPTOMS

Prodrome

☐ Mood changes ☐ Food cravings ☐ Yawning ☐ Thirst

☐ Frequent urination ☐ Fatigue ☐ Neck stiffness

☐ Concentration ☐ Smell sensitive ☐ Other: ____________________

Aura

☐ Visual changes ☐ Numbness/tingling ☐ Speech difficulty

☐ Weakness ☐ Dizziness ☐ Other: ____________________

HEADACHE PHASE

Pain location

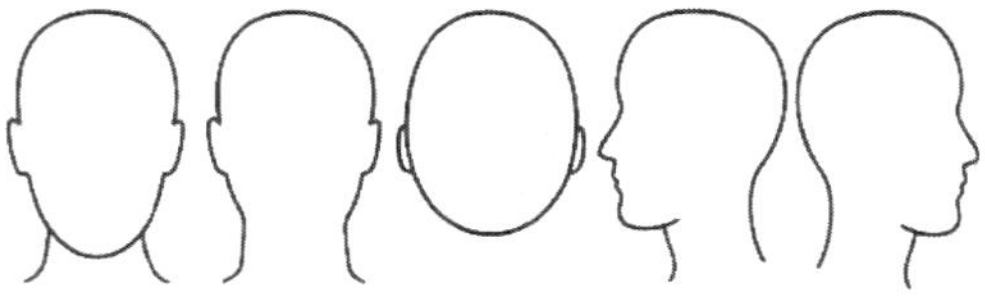

FRONT BACK TOP LEFT RIGHT

Pain quality:

☐ Throbbing ☐ Pressure

☐ Stabbing ☐ Burning

☐ Tight ☐ Other:

Intensity: 0 1 2 3 4 5

Other symptoms:

☐ Nausea ☐ Vomiting ☐ Dizziness ☐ Fatigue

☐ Confusion ☐ Neck pain ☐ Vision changes ☐ Anxiety

☐ Light sensitivity ☐ Sound sensitivity ☐ Smell sensitivity ☐ Skin sensitivity

☐ Other:

TRIGGERS

Tick any factors you believe/suspect contributed to this episode, even if you also tracked them in your monthly log.

☐ Stress/emotion ☐ Food/drink ☐ Weather/environment

☐ Exercise/activity ☐ Hormonal ☐ Screen time

☐ Other:

RELIEF STRATEGIES & MEDICATIONS USED

List medications and non-medication strategies (rest, dark room, cold/heat packs, hydration, sleep, relaxation techniques, etc.

Time (approx.)	Medication/ Strategy	Effective? (1 no relief-5 complete)	Side Effects	Rebound Y/N

RESOLUTION AND POSTDROME

End Date: / / Time ____________ Total Duration ____________

How it ended

☐ Gradual ☐ Sudden ☐ Other

Postdrome Symptoms

☐ Fatigue ☐ Confusion ☐ Mood changes

☐ Head pain with movement ☐ Light/sound sensitivity

☐ Other:

Impact:

Missed activities, work, social plans?

NOTES: Unusual symptoms, suspected new triggers, reflections, etc.

____

____

____

Section 3 Reflection and Support

Tracking is most useful when you take time to look back at what you've recorded. This section helps you reflect on the strategies you've tried, the self-care practices that support you, and the patterns you've noticed. It also gives space for personal notes and to bring everything together in your migraine journey.

While the earlier sections focus on daily and monthly details, these pages are about stepping back to see the bigger picture. Reflection can highlight progress you may not have noticed in the moment and point to small changes that could help in the future.

You do not need to write a lot. Simple notes on what worked, what didn't, and what you'd like to try next can be enough to guide your next steps. These reflections are for your personal insight and to support more focused conversations with your healthcare provider.

Looking back on your records can show you details you might otherwise overlook. Even brief notes can highlight patterns worth paying attention to.

Preventative Strategies to Try

Use this page to list new approaches you want to explore. Add who suggested them, why you want to try them, and what you expect. After trying, rate how effective it was on a scale of 1 to 5, where 1 is 'not effective' to 5 'highly effective'.

Strategy Categories

These are examples of possible strategies and the list is not exhaustive. Add your own ideas as you experiment with your migraine management.

- Sleep routines – keeping regular bedtimes, wake times, naps.
- Nutrition & hydration – adjusting diet, meal timing, water intake.
- Stress management – therapy, journaling, setting boundaries.
- Physical activity – gentle movement, yoga, strength training.
- Environmental & sensory adjustments – lighting, noise, air quality, screen time.
- Relaxation techniques – breathing, meditation, massage, stretching.
- Support systems – friends, family, workplace accommodations, peer groups.
- Lifestyle balance – pacing activities, planning breaks, managing workload.
- Medical / professional support – preventive meds, physiotherapy, acupuncture, CBT, biofeedback.
- Trigger awareness – reducing or avoiding personal migraine triggers.

Strategy	Suggested By	Expected Benefits	Effectiveness and Notes
Magnesium supplement	Doctor	Suggested it may reduce migraine frequency	3. Took daily for 2 months, it helped a little

Strategy	Suggested By	Expected Benefits	Effectiveness and Notes

Strategy	Suggested By	Expected Benefits	Effectiveness and Notes

Self-Care Strategies

These pages help you build your personal self-care toolkit, the things that make you feel more balanced and resilient. Unlike preventive strategies, which you might be experimenting with, this section is about capturing what consistently supports you. Rate the helpfulness on a scale of 1 (not helpful) to 5 (very helpful). This tracker is designed to help you identify patterns and track your experiences. Small, consistent changes often have the biggest impact on your overall well-being.

Tip: Check back against your migraine and stress trackers to see how self-care practices line up with better or worse days.

Key Areas for Self-Care with Examples

- Sleep – regular bedtime, quality rest, naps when needed.
- Hydration & Nutrition – water goals, balanced meals, avoiding skipped meals.
- Stress Management – journaling, therapy, breathing practices, setting boundaries.
- Physical Well-being – stretching, gentle exercise, movement breaks, posture.
- Environmental Factors – quiet spaces, natural light, reducing clutter or noise.
- Social Support – connection with friends, family, peer groups, asking for help.
- Lifestyle Balance – pacing activities, planning downtime, managing workload.
- Meaning & Purpose – meditation, values, spiritual or reflective practices.

Strategy	Date	Helpfulness and Notes
10-minute stretching before bed	10 March	5. Relaxing, better sleep, reduced morning tension.

Strategy	Date	Helpfulness and Notes

Strategy	Date	Helpfulness and Notes

Which self-care strategies made the biggest difference to you?

My Migraine Journey

This section helps you bring everything together: what you've learned from tracking, the patterns you've noticed, and the strategies you've tried that have made a difference. It's also a space to prepare for future conversations with your healthcare providers and to set intentions for the next stage of your migraine management.

My most effective treatments are

Early warning signs I've identified

Lifestyle changes that have helped

Questions for My Doctor/Healthcare Provider

As you track your migraines, new questions can come up. Note them here so you can remember them for your next appointment.

Progress and Next Steps

Tracker end date: / / 20

Use this page to bring together what stood out during this tracking period and what you want to carry into the next one. Note the patterns that matter most, strategies worth continuing, and the directions you'd like to explore further.

Key patterns to continue monitoring

Treatments to explore

What helped most

Next steps in my migraine management

Personal Notes & Observations

Use these pages for any additional thoughts, observations, or patterns you notice.

GLOSSARY

Acute Treatment (also called rescue treatment)

A medication or strategy used during a migraine attack to reduce pain or symptoms (for example, triptans, NSAIDs, rest, cold packs).

Allodynia

Pain or discomfort caused by normally non-painful touch or pressure (such as brushing hair or wearing glasses).

Aura

Neurological symptoms that may occur before or during a migraine. These can include visual changes (flashing lights, zig-zag lines, blind spots), numbness or tingling, speech difficulty, or dizziness. Aura usually lasts from a few minutes to an hour.

Chronic Migraine

A form of migraine where headache occurs on 15 or more days per month, with at least 8 of those days having migraine-specific features.

Episode Log

A detailed record of a single migraine attack, including early symptoms, headache phase, treatments used, and recovery.

Headache Phase

The stage of migraine when pain is present. Pain is often throbbing or pulsing, can affect one or both sides of the head, and may worsen with movement, light, or sound.

Hormonal Migraine

Migraine linked to hormonal changes, often occurring around menstruation, ovulation, pregnancy, or menopause.

Medication Codes

Shorthand labels used in the monthly tracker to record which medications were taken. For example, R1 or R2 for prescription medications, and O1, O2, O3 for over-the-counter medications. A key at the bottom of each tracker page lets you define what each code means.

Menstrual Migraine

Migraine attacks that occur in relation to menstruation, typically in the two days before bleeding begins and the first three days of the period.

Migraine Day

Any day on which migraine symptoms are present. For tracking purposes, this usually means days where headache severity is 2 or higher on a 0–5 scale, or days where migraine-specific symptoms (aura, nausea, light sensitivity) are present.

NSAIDs

Non-steroidal anti-inflammatory drugs, a group of pain relievers often used for migraine. Examples include ibuprofen and naproxen.

Postdrome

The recovery stage after the headache pain eases. Sometimes called a "migraine hangover." Symptoms may include fatigue, confusion, sensitivity to light or sound, or mood changes. This phase can last hours to a couple of days.

Preventive Treatment

Medication or lifestyle strategies used regularly to reduce how often or how severe migraine attacks are.

Prodrome

The early warning phase that occurs hours or even days before migraine pain begins. Symptoms may include mood changes, food cravings, yawning, fatigue, neck stiffness, or difficulty concentrating.

Recurrence

When migraine pain returns within 24 hours after initial relief from treatment.

Supplements

Vitamins, minerals, herbal remedies, or other non-prescription substances taken to support health or migraine management.

Threshold

The point at which several small factors build up and trigger a migraine attack. For example, lack of sleep, stress, and certain foods may combine to cross a personal threshold.

Treatment effect codes

Abbreviations used in the monthly tracker to show how well a treatment worked.
S = Success (complete relief), P = Partial (some relief), F = Fail (no relief),
* = Recurred (worked at first but migraine returned within 24 hours).

Triggers

Factors that can increase the chance of a migraine attack. Common triggers include stress, sleep changes, certain foods or drinks, hormonal shifts, weather changes, or prolonged screen time.

Thank You

Thank you for using this Migraine Tracker. We hope it has helped you notice patterns and gather useful information about your migraines.

This book is not a medical tool and does not replace professional advice. Please continue to share what you've tracked with your healthcare provider and use it as a starting point for those conversations.

If this tracker has supported you in any way, please leave a review on Amazon. Even a brief comment makes a difference and helps more people living with migraines find the resources they need.

Remember: managing migraines is an ongoing process. Every note you make adds to your understanding and can help guide your next steps. Keep this tracker for reference when you begin your next tracking period.

About Book & Bat Publishing

Book & Bat Publishing creates practical guides, journals, and workbooks designed to make life a little easier and more manageable. Our focus is always on clarity, usefulness, and accessibility. In other words, books you can pick up and start using straight away, without overwhelm or jargon.

Our catalogue ranges from self-care journals and values workbooks to tools for decluttering, ADHD support, and emotional wellbeing. Whatever the topic, our authors make sure that every Book & Bat Publishing title is built to give readers confidence and practical steps they can trust.

Found This Book Helpful?

If this book helped you, please consider leaving a short review on Amazon. Your review makes a big difference, it helps others find the support they need and helps us keep creating useful, grounded resources.

Thank you for reading. We hope these tools make a real difference in your work life.

If you'd like us to tell you when we publish our next book, please join our mailing list at www.bookandbat.com or scan the QR code.

You Might Also Be Interested In

365 Self-Care Activities for Women

365 Self-Care Activities for Women offers a full year of simple, practical ideas to nurture your wellbeing every day.

The Core Values Workbook

A guided workbook to help you identify, understand, and apply your personal values in everyday decisions and relationships.

Breathwork Essentials

Simple, effective breathing techniques to calm your nervous system and reset in the moment — no experience needed.

Executive Function for Adults with ADHD

Clear, practical tools to manage time, focus, organization, and follow-through. Written for real life, not perfection.

Navigating Anxious Attachment

Grounded support for building emotional safety, managing overthinking, and creating secure connections.

Navigating Avoidant Attachment

A practical guide for understanding emotional distancing, reconnecting with your needs, and building trust without overwhelm.

To explore more practical tools from Book & Bat Publishing, visit www.bookandbat.com/books.

Made in United States
North Haven, CT
05 November 2026

21767740R10072